Your
Sexual
Health

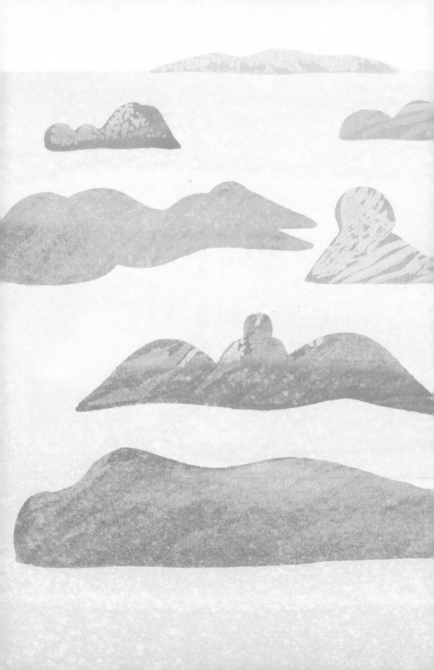

Kate White, M.D.

Your Sexual Health

A Guide to Understanding,
Loving and Caring for Your Body

Illustrations by Monica Ramos

MAYO CLINIC PRESS

Introduction

Afterword

Introduction

Growing up, my body below my waist was a mystery. I went to Catholic school until I was 12, and my public schools weren't much better at teaching me the things I needed to know about sexual health. I didn't know what vaginal discharge was, so was horrified to see wetness on my underwear at age 14 and worried I was peeing myself. My well-meaning mother told me in college that oral sex was perverted. It wasn't until medical school that I finally learned the basics (and then some) about my reproductive health.

You shouldn't have to go to medical school to learn the fundamentals about your body. But where else can you get sexual health knowledge? The internet is a mixed bag of the good, the bad and the intentionally misleading. Unlike your doctor, your search engine isn't board-certified to practice medicine. If you're turning to your siblings and friends for insights, they usually don't have access to information that's any better than you can find (despite how confidently they may give you advice). Even savvy, smart people have been confused by misinformation or conflicting recommendations.

Maybe you know the basics but want more details about how your private parts work and how best to use them. You can find yourself lost trying to get the knowledge you need to make the best choices about your health. It's tough to find good information about sex toys because they make some people blush or giggle. Or about how birth control affects your periods, because the glossy pamphlets you get in the doctor's office are a sales pitch. Or about abortion because it's so politically charged. And you'll rarely see a doctor's office brochure about anal sex.

That's why I wrote this book.

Your Sexual Health is full of the critical knowledge and secrets I've learned from being an obstetrician-gynecologist and a health writer for more than 20 years. This book offers answers to the questions patients and reporters have asked me repeatedly — and the questions you've maybe been too embarrassed to ask. The information in this book will help you make solid decisions, feel less anxious and control your reproductive destiny. Consider this book your crash course in better sexual health.

> **Note: This book is intended for people with a vagina, of any identity or orientation. Gendered language and references to hetero or lesbian women reflect the limitations of published research that hasn't that hasn't caught up to the times.**

Part I. Gyno Health

The land down under

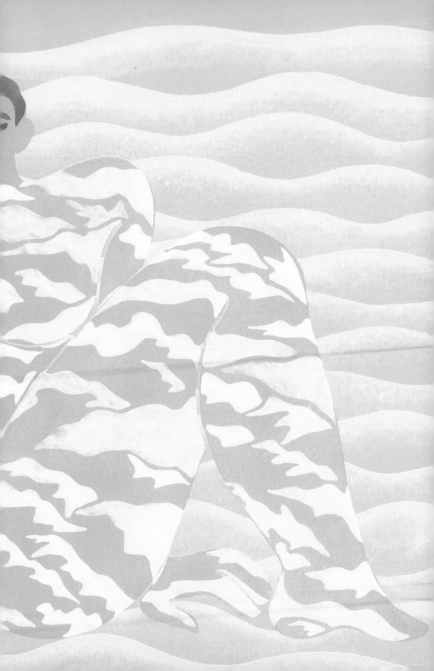

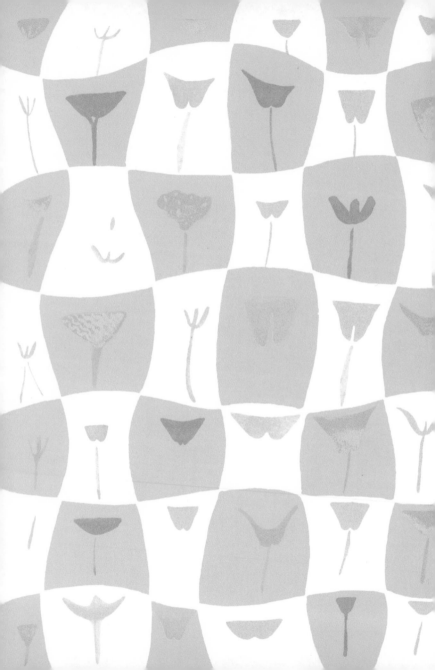

1. You may be calling your parts by the wrong names.

2. Your labia are normal, no matter how long or short they are.

3. Your vagina should smell (and taste) like a vagina.

4. Protect your parts, not your panties.

5. Douching your discharge is dangerous.

6. All that itches isn't yeast.

7. Waxing won't give you herpes — but your skin may look like it does.

8. Never go back to front.

9. Treat your vulva like the Hope Diamond.

10. (Almost) everyone gets HPV at some point.

11. You don't need a yearly Pap, but an annual visit is a good idea.

12. An abnormal Pap doesn't mean you have cancer.

13. We don't care if you've shaved.

14. If you don't feel comfortable talking to your gyno, find another one.

15. We *want* to hear about your sex life.

1 You may be calling your parts by the wrong names.

You'll hear the word *vagina* used to refer to the genitals of a person assigned female at birth. The vagina is an amazing organ—it can stretch to accommodate nearly anything that's put inside it, and almost any baby on its way out. But the vagina is *inside* the body. The only way you can see the vagina is with a speculum and a hand mirror.

The part of the anatomy you *can* easily see is the vulva. Your vulva begins at the clitoris and the skin (hood) covering it. Packed with nerve endings, this is the most sensitive spot on your body, and the only human organ dedicated purely to pleasure. The vulva then extends down to your perineum, the skin and muscle in between the opening of your vagina and your anus.

In between, you have two sets of lips (labia). The outer set is called the labia majora. This is what forms a cameltoe when you wear tight clothing. The inner set is called the labia minora and can be pierced if you're adventurous. Go to MayoClinic.org and search on *vulva* to get a closer look at all the parts described here.

Knowing what's where will help you understand how your body behaves—and help you talk with your gyno when something seems funky.

Your labia are normal, no matter how long or short they are.

2

Genitals come in an array of shapes, sizes and colors. Some people have thin labia (minora) that extend out beyond the plump ones (majora). Other people's thin labia are totally covered. No matter what you may have seen in porn or on a partner, yours are just fine.

Unethical doctors will prey on people's body insecurity and offer them cosmetic surgery for their labia so they can match up to some mythical ideal. But there are only two indications for someone to take a scalpel to your nether region: for gender reassignment/realignment, or if your labia are long enough to cause pain with intercourse or tight clothing. Otherwise, accept your labia like you do the rest of your body, in all its quirky wonder.

And in case you're wondering about how a partner may view your body? Any partner who sees you naked should count their lucky stars that they get to be that close to you, first and foremost. If your partner has anything to say about your labia — or any other part of your body — that's not akin to ecstatic worship, it's time to trade up to someone worthy of you.

3 Your vagina should smell (and taste) like a vagina.

Not berries, flowers or a tropical island. You have a naturally musky, pheromone-filled scent. And the taste of your vagina varies depending on where you are in your cycle — muskier around ovulation, and metallic-tinged when you're bleeding. Attempting to cover up your scent with sprays and powders may trigger irritation of the vulva and vagina (contact dermatitis) and lead to more discharge and possibly an infection. What about those blogs that tell you to eat pineapples or avoid asparagus to improve the way you taste? There's no science that proves there's a relationship between your diet and your taste or odor.

If you notice a strange odor, particularly a fishy one, have your gyno check you out for a vaginal infection. Your gyno can take a simple swab of your vagina, and you'll have results in 24–48 hours. Otherwise, you smell and taste just the way you should. And any partner who has a problem with the way your vagina (naturally) smells or tastes should lose the privilege to be anywhere near one.

Protect your parts, not your panties.

4

It's not uncommon to be bothered by vaginal discharge — it's one of the most common reasons for a gyno visit. When people don't like the feeling of moisture on their underwear, they may use a pantiliner every day. But blocking your vagina with a pad is the worst thing you can do. When your vagina can't breathe, it may react by producing even *more* discharge. This can happen even with reusable liners. Plus, tossing all those disposable liners is rotten for the environment. Save the liners for light period days.

If your panties get wet, simply change them. The reason we wear underwear is to protect our clothes. You shouldn't use liners to protect your underwear. If you're out and about, bring along a spare pair of underwear in a plastic bag. When you're ready to swap, just zip the old ones into the bag. Easy-peasy.

5 Douching your discharge is dangerous.

A vagina naturally has discharge — same goes for many trans-women's vaginas after gender affirmation surgery. Discharge is how your vagina cleans itself, keeps the tissue moist, gets you ready for intercourse and helps prevent infection. Think of it as daily intimate housekeeping. Your discharge should be clear, white, or off-white, though it varies in amount and consistency at different times in your cycle, at different ages, and if you're on certain medications.

Wash only your vulva, with your fingers, water and a gentle soap. Don't interfere with your body's self-cleaning by putting soap or a washcloth *into* the vagina. And above all, **do not douche,** which is cleaning out the inside of the vagina with water, either alone or mixed, with other fluids. Douches are often sold in a bottle or bag, and you're meant to squirt the fluids upward through a tube or nozzle into your vagina.

Exposing the vulva to chemicals and perfumes increases your risk of irritation and infection.

Even a baking-soda-only douche pushes bacteria from your vagina up into your uterus, where they don't belong. This can cause pelvic inflammatory disease. And there's no such thing as a "natural" douche — there's no "safe alternative." Bottom line: Your body knows how to clean itself. Let it do its thing.

All that itches isn't yeast.

6

Many people assume that itching on the vulva means a yeast infection and immediately buy a drugstore treatment or start scarfing yogurt to fix it. But different vaginal infections can be mistaken for one another, and each needs different treatment.

Yeast infections tend to come with a thick, white, cottage-cheese-type discharge. If you have a discharge that looks like curdled milk and you can't stop scratching, a drugstore treatment is worth a try.

Yogurt won't treat a yeast infection, whether you eat it or put it in your vagina (and please don't do that).

You may also get itchy with a bacterial vaginosis (BV) infection. BV is an overgrowth of bacteria that naturally live in your vagina. This infection can have a thicker, sometimes yellow discharge, and an unpleasant "fishy" odor. The difference in discharge can help you figure out which infection you might have. But even doctors are lousy at identifying an infection just by looking in your vagina.

If your over-the-counter treatment for a yeast infection isn't making you feel much better in three days, head to the gyno's office for a test to figure out what's going on.

7 Waxing won't give you herpes — but your skin may look like it does.

My patient had a full Brazilian wax before a dream trip to Greece. When she returned, she was terrified that her hot Grecian hook-up gave her herpes. She was thrilled to hear that it wasn't herpes, but folliculitis — an irritation and infection of the hair follicles caused by waxing or shaving. These angry red bumps can be painful or itchy and can look like herpes. Here's how to know the difference: A herpes outbreak, especially if it's your first, is extremely painful. You may also have a fever and swollen lymph nodes in your groin. Herpes can appear on your labia and inside the vagina.

How can you prevent folliculitis? If you wax, use a fresh jar of wax that wasn't used for anyone else. If you shave, change your razor more often than you do now. Old razors develop nicks in the blades that can cause tiny tears in your skin and put you at risk of an infection. If you're prone to razor burn, buy cheap single-blade razors in bulk (or refillable blade cartridges) and toss them after each use. It may seem awful for the environment, but it's healthier for your skin. If you get folliculitis, topical hydrocortisone cream can speed healing.

Never go back to front.

8

This goes for wiping and for having sex. Wiping back to front after using the loo brings unhealthy bacteria from your anus into your vagina and sets you up for a bladder infection. People with vaginas are prone to these infections, also known as urinary tract infections (UTIs). Since the passageway leading into the bladder (urethra) is so short, compared to how long it is in a penis, it's easy for bacteria to climb up. No matter how quickly you're trying to get out of the rest-room, make sure to wipe from front to back. Always.

> **When you can, drink a full glass of water and pee after intercourse. This lowers your risk of UTIs even further.**

Having vaginal intercourse right after anal intercourse poses the same risks. Anal play should be the last thing you do during a sex session. If you change your mind during sex and want to keep playing after anal, make sure your partner washes up — with water *and* soap — before heading back to you. Same goes for sex toys.

9 Treat your vulva like the Hope Diamond.

It may not sparkle in quite the same way (and I definitely don't recommend "vajazzling"), but it's just as valuable, and you have only one. Treat it with care. That means no harsh chemicals on your nether regions. No perfumed sprays, no douches. Be cautious even with scented pantiliners. In the shower or bath, puffs and washcloths may be too abrasive for such delicate skin. And if you're dealing with lots of vaginal discharge, use the mildest soap and laundry detergent possible. I like the formulations meant for babies, but any fragrance-free detergent is a good choice.

Let your vulva see the light of day from time to time. Go to bed without panties, even if you're alone, to let your vulva and vagina breathe. Don't like sleeping naked? Going bare under boxers or a nightshirt does the same thing. Change out of wet bathing suits or workout gear as soon as you can, especially if they're nylon. And go commando if you're feeling frisky and it's context-appropriate.

10 (Almost) everyone gets HPV at some point.

You've probably heard of human papillomavirus (HPV), and how it's the cause of most cancers of the cervix (and vagina and vulva). But you might not know how common HPV infection is. At any given time, about 42 million people are infected with HPV and may not even know it.

> **HPV is so common that nearly *all* sexually active women, men and nonbinary folks get the virus at some point in their lives.**

The good news is that most HPV infections clear on their own or become undetectable, and most infections never lead to disease (such as genital warts or changing cervical cells). If you're under 30, you're even more likely to clear your HPV infection on your own. If you're a tobacco smoker, here's another good reason to quit: If you do, your HPV infection will likely resolve faster.

The best way to prevent HPV is with the vaccine, available at your doctor's office or pharmacy that offers vaccinations. Everyone from age 11 to 26, no matter their gender identity, should get the vaccine series. Some people older than that — age 27 to 45 — may benefit, and they should talk with their doctor. Even if you've had HPV in the past, the vaccine prevents getting infected with *other* strains that put you at risk of cancer. Beyond that, using external or internal condoms every time you have intercourse can reduce your risk of HPV infection. Notice I said "reduce." Since HPV lives in the skin of your genitals, rubbing up against your partner — during intercourse or at any other time — can transmit an HPV infection.

If you get diagnosed with HPV, should you tell your partner(s)? The answer to that question is an unequivocal yes for every *other* sexually transmitted infection. But it's a bit tricky with HPV. Partners with penises can't be tested for the virus, and no one can be treated for the infection (except for the removal of genital warts or cervical cells if needed). And you'll never know who gave the infection to whom. So, while I recommend honesty in all things sexual, you can be forgiven for not talking to your partner about your HPV infection. If you do decide to talk about it, come with information from your gyno or the Centers for Disease Control and Prevention (CDC) about how common the infection is, and how you both likely have it. You can also have your partner follow up with a doctor — or hand over this book.

11 You don't need a yearly Pap, but an annual visit is a good idea.

Doctors have figured out that people (especially young people) were getting Paps too often. Yes, there's such a thing as too much testing. Doctors started to detect abnormalities of the cervix that would have resolved on their own if they'd been left alone. All this testing meant that too many people were subjected to unnecessary and painful treatment, which for some led to complications with childbirth later. So, good news: No Paps until you turn 21, then every three to five years after that, depending on if your gyno can also test for HPV at the same time. (Different rules apply if you've had an abnormal Pap at some point.)

Even if you're not sexually active with partners with a penis, you still need to get regular Paps.

But don't skip the annual exam completely. I tell my patients, "You're more than just a cervix to me." An annual visit is a great chance to talk with your gyno about any pelvic and sexual health concerns, lets you get checked for sexually transmitted infections (STIs) and gives you an opportunity to review birth control options. You may even be able to keep your pants on (what a relief).

An abnormal Pap doesn't mean you have cancer.

12

If you get a letter from your doctor's office or see your actual test results, Pap test language can be terrifying. "Low grade squamous intraepithelial lesion," "undetermined significance," "atypical glandular cells" — it's no wonder my office gets calls from panicked patients who don't know what their results mean. Pap tests offer a detailed look at the cells on your cervix. They can detect many different types of changes *years* before cervical cancer develops.

If you have an abnormal Pap test (including a positive HPV result), your gyno will recommend one of three things: stay on your normal testing schedule (because there's no cause for concern), repeat the Pap in one year, or come in for a detailed exam of your cervix called a colposcopy. Your gyno will apply one of two solutions (vinegar or iodine-based) to your cervix and take samples from any areas that look even remotely suspicious (a biopsy). (Side note: Ask if you can cough when this is done — it helps with the pain.)

You may have more testing or treatment based on the results of the colposcopy and biopsies. If you follow your gyno's recommendations, the chances of you developing cancer are slim.

13 We don't care if you've shaved.

Many of my patients apologize before their pelvic exam for not shaving, waxing or somehow "prepping" for their visit. Some are concerned that hair is going to get in the way of an exam of their skin. Or worried that the speculum will snag their hair on the way out or in. Or — let's be honest — they're worried that they're not conforming to some beauty standard that they think they need to live up to, even at the doctor's office.

I can tell you that gynos are so focused on your exam and making sure that you're healthy, that we don't notice what your hair looks like down there. As for your hair getting in the way of the exam or the speculum? Your gyno knows how to work around anything that gets in the way of the vagina, be it hair, long labia, or restricted movement of your legs. Your exam will be just fine.

Don't jump to cancelling your exam if you're on your period. We don't care if you're bleeding, and we can still perform most testing. If you're not sure if you should reschedule your appointment, call your doctor's office.

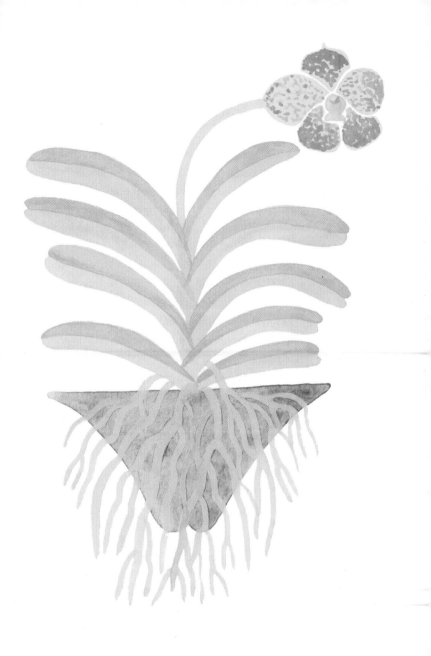

14 If you don't feel comfortable talking to your gyno, find another one.

Your health is too important to not discuss it with your doctor. You should feel as comfortable talking about sex and periods and birth control with your gyno as you do hanging out with your friends. And since about half of women will have urinary leakage (incontinence) during their lives, which includes some women under 40, you need someone you can talk to. Your gyno is likely better-informed than your buddies and can give you advice targeted to your specific needs, unlike the internet. If you're worried about bringing up certain topics with a doctor that you might have been going to since you were a teen (anal sex! decreased libido! trouble getting pregnant!), don't worry — we've heard it all.

And if you *do* bring up your deepest fears with your doctor and you're met with anything other than empathy and advice, move on. There are plenty of great gynos out there. No one should put up with rushing or judgment from their health care provider. If you're super-limited in where you can get care and you're striking out finding a good gyno, try a family medicine doctor or a nurse practitioner.

We *want* to hear about your sex life. 15

Not because we're nosy or hungry for gossip. But because between nearly half of women report problems with sexual desire, arousal or orgasm to us at some point. And because pain with sex is common — and not just when it's your first time. Because you may be struggling with your sexual feelings and feeling constricted because of the culture or religion you grew up in. Because you might have been assaulted at some point, and you might need to talk about it. Because if you're not feeling safe in your relationship, we can give you resources and help you plan. Because you may be exploring your sexual identity or your gender identity, and we want to be a safe place where you can talk about it and give you good information. We want our office to be a safe space for you to tell us about your sex life. It's not an overshare.

Your doctor will likely ask you if you're having any concerns about sex. But if we don't ask, I hope you'll feel free to tell — it's the only way we can help.

Body Checkup

Check in with yourself by answering these questions:

- ☐ Is my vaginal discharge amount, color and odor normal for me, or does something seem off?
- ☐ Do I feel the need to douche or to use pantiliners when I'm not bleeding?
- ☐ Do I often get bumps after shaving or waxing?
- ☐ Am I up to date on my Pap test?
- ☐ Have I been fully vaccinated against HPV?
- ☐ Have I been checked for sexually transmitted infections in the past year?
- ☐ Can I be fully open with my gyno about my sex life?

Ask Your Doctor...

I encourage you to ask your doctor any of these questions:

- ☐ Can I swab myself to check for STIs or vaginal infection?
- ☐ Can you tell if my vaginal discharge is OK, or if it's a sign I have an infection?
- ☐ What do my Pap test results mean?
- ☐ When I get my Pap, do you test me for HPV at the same time? If you don't, when do I need to get a test for HPV?
- ☐ How often should I get a Pap test?
- ☐ Do I have to have a pelvic exam if I'm feeling fine?

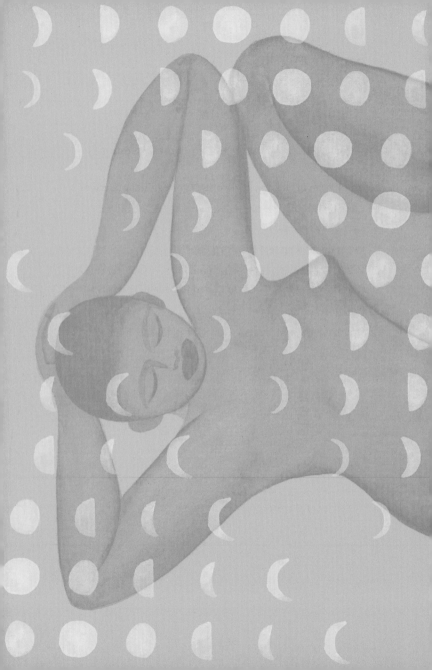

Bleed, rinse, repeat

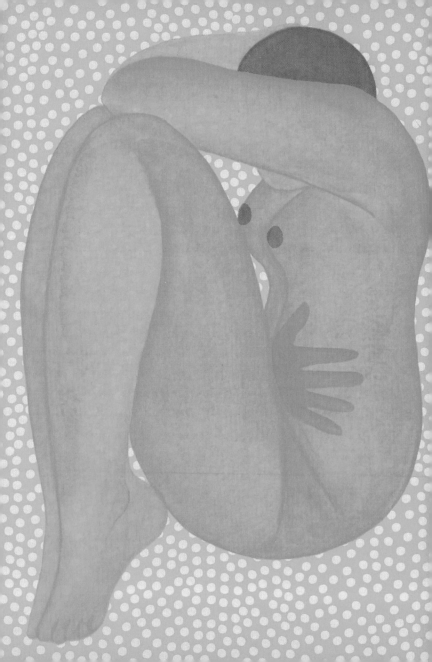

16. It's normal to not be normal sometimes.

17. What you think "regular" means is different from what your gyno thinks it means.

18. There's more to period products than tampons and pads.

19. Your periods will change throughout your life.

20. You're not going to get toxic shock.

21. There's no totally safe time to have sex and not get pregnant.

22. You don't have to live with heavy periods.

23. You don't have to live with pain during periods.

24. You don't have to live with PMS.

25. Listen to your gut (and your uterus).

16 It's normal to not be normal sometimes.

Beyond changes in timing, periods can change in character. Some months your period may last only three to four days, then occasionally you're bleeding for a week. You may get random spotting in the middle of a cycle, which may catch you by surprise. And sometimes your period may ghost you completely. Think of your period as having a flaky personality.

Stick liners in all your bags so that you're ready for the unexpected.

In certain times of your life, your periods may get incredibly heavy. When you're under a great deal of stress, for example, your periods can reflect your emotional state. When you're transitioning back to normal periods after a pregnancy, your periods can be irregular or heavy. Some medications can change your period. So can switching your hormonal birth control. And many things can cause a late or missed period, including stress, illness and travel.

How abnormal is *too* abnormal? Head to your gyno if you have spotting more months than you don't, your periods routinely last more than a week, or your bleeding becomes so heavy that you're changing your period products every two hours or have clots larger than a grape. And while it's normal to skip a period once in a while, talk to your gyno if you're not having a period at least once every few months. It's good to know what's going on with your body.

A healthy kind of "not normal" is when you're using hormonal birth control. When you're using contraception such as the pill, patch or ring, you have lighter-than-normal (and less-crampy) periods. In fact, the bleeding you see at the end of each month isn't really a period. It's a *withdrawal bleed* that occurs from the sudden stop of hormones during the placebo week of pills or patch- or ring-free week. Fun fact: Birth control was designed to have a withdrawal bleed because researchers thought this regimen would be acceptable to the Pope, as it seemed like a natural variant of the "rhythm" method of birth control.

Even skipping your "period" on birth control completely is perfectly healthy. The hormones in contraception keep the lining of your uterus so thin that sometimes you don't bleed at all. Many birth control methods can help you achieve period-free living. You can use birth control pills continuously by skipping the placebo pills, and you can use the monthly rings back-to-back. You may also see no bleeding with certain IUDs, the implant or the injection. If you have nightmarish periods — heavy bleeding or cramping, or miserable PMS — not having them at all could be life-changing.

17 What you think "regular" means is different from what your gyno thinks it means.

Many patients tell me they have "irregular periods." But when they describe their periods, their patterns sound typical to me.

Menstruating people often expect to have periods that start on the same day of each month or think their periods should come like clockwork every 28 days. Then when their menstrual patterns look uneven on their phone tracker, they think they have irregular periods.

Very few people have 28-day cycles every month. It's much more common to have cycles that vary in length.

Counting from the first day of bleeding one month to the first day of bleeding in the next month, your gyno is expecting your cycle to land in the 21- to 35-day range. You may get the occasional 28-day cycle, but more commonly, your cycles will vary in length. So, it can be hard to say exactly when your next period is going to start. But as far as your gyno is concerned, "about monthly" is regular enough for us.

What is *too* irregular? If your periods generally come more often than every three weeks or less often than every five weeks, check with your gyno. Very irregular periods may be a sign of hormone issues or polycystic ovary syndrome.

There's more to period products than tampons and pads.

18

People with periods used to have just two choices: pads or tampons. Disposable pads can cause chafing and are terrible for the environment, and many people are concerned about the chemicals in the cotton used for tampons.

Now the menses marketplace is full of options: organic pads, menstrual cups and discs, reusable cotton pads and period underwear. If you're irritated by your pads or leaking through a tampon and need a combination of products, or you just want something more environmentally friendly, you can shop around.

The downside of some of these choices? They're not cheap. A menstrual cup can run you $35, and a single pair of period underwear can cost nearly $50. Of course, a reusable product will cost less than disposable ones over time, but the upfront cost may be too much.

Before you plunk down the money, think about what it might be like to use a new product. Do you work in an office where changing a full menstrual cup might be challenging in a shared restroom? Do you have easy access to laundry for reusable products — or a mesh bag where you can store the used ones until laundry day? Check out online reviews and ask friends about their experiences.

19 Your periods will change throughout your life.

Very few people who have periods will have the same kind of bleeding pattern from middle school through middle age. For most people, their very first period will be light, short and brown in color. In those first few years of bleeding, periods are often random, and it's not uncommon to skip them sometimes. Early periods vary in flow, too, with some light and some super-heavy. After a time, most people find that their periods settle into a relatively predictable rhythm.

This pattern may change if you get pregnant, but some people find that their periods become fairly regular again after a pregnancy. And pain with periods may actually improve after having a baby. As you enter your 40s, it's not uncommon for your last few years of bleeding to be like your first years — unpredictable, heavy and brown once again.

Knowing that your menstrual cycle will change over time may be a source of comfort. If your periods are miserable right now, for instance, give it a few years and it may change on its own. (Though if your periods are making you miserable, talk to your gyno. We can help make them better.)

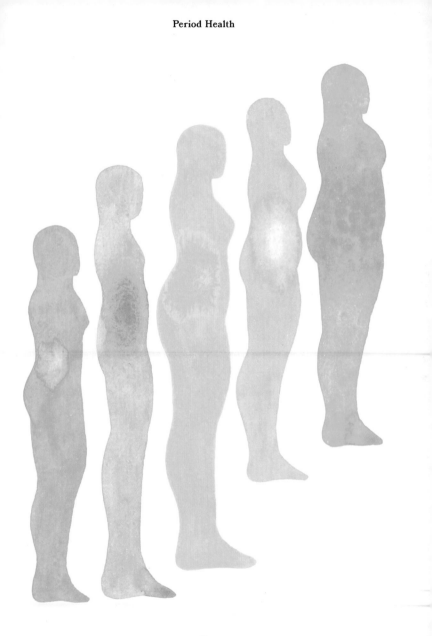

20 You're not going to get toxic shock.

Growing up, my friends were terrified of using tampons. Not because they didn't want to put them inside their bodies, but because they were afraid of toxic shock syndrome (TSS). TSS is a serious infection that starts in the vagina and spreads throughout the body. It happens when menstrual blood is allowed to stay in the body for a long time. In effect, the bloody tampon acts like a petri dish for a bacterial infection to grow and spread. Gross and scary, right?

While TSS *can* happen, it's important to put the risk in perspective. The average menstruating woman has less than a 1-in-100,000 chance of developing toxic shock. That means you're as likely to die from TSS as you are to die in a plane crash or while skydiving or at a dance party. Plus, you can avoid TSS by simply changing your tampon every four to eight hours, and by not using more absorbency than you need. If tampons are your preferred menstrual product, you can use them without worry.

Menstrual cup fans can get TSS, too. However, only five cases have ever been reported. But the same advice holds for anything in your vagina during your periods: Don't leave your menstrual cup in too long. Look to the instructions that come with your menstrual cup for guidance.

There's no totally safe time to have sex and not get pregnant.

21

"You can't get pregnant during your period" is a myth. The logic is alluring: If you have sex during your period, then you're far away from the middle of your cycle when your ovaries release an egg. That timing should keep you safe, right?

Not necessarily. First, sperm are hardy creatures. They can live up to five days, waiting for an egg to appear. While menstrual cycles last 28 days on average, if you have a shorter cycle one month, sperm could live long enough to fertilize the egg. Plus, not all vaginal bleeding is your period. Even if you bleed like clockwork, you may have an episode of heavy spotting that you mistake for a period. When that happens, your mental math gets thrown off, and you could end up having sex right when you're ovulating.

Fertility awareness methods of birth control can help you avoid getting pregnant by identifying the days in your cycle when pregnancy is possible. However, it's possible for these days to overlap with a period, especially if your periods aren't regular. This is why about 1 out of 4 people using this method will get pregnant each year. *Anytime* you have unprotected sex with a sperm-producing partner, you may get pregnant.

22 You don't have to live with heavy periods.

Most menstruators aren't fond of their periods. Sure, it means your system is working as it's meant to, but it can be a drag dealing with bleeding during white-pants season, if you're swimming, or if you're sexually active with a partner. For some people, bleeding is so heavy that it impacts every part of their lives. I've had patients report bleeding onto car seats and bed sheets and desk chairs, so much that they're afraid to leave the house when bleeding is the worst. Some people bleed so much that they sit on the toilet so they can bleed right into the bowl on their heavy flow days.

What do doctors consider heavy bleeding? Periods that routinely last more than seven days, need more than five menstrual products in a day, or cause bleeding through your clothes. Talk to a gyno about figuring out why this is happening. Your doctor may recommend blood tests, ultrasounds, or a biopsy of the lining of your uterus. If your gyno finds something in your uterus like a polyp or fibroid, it can be removed. If you have a hormonal imbalance, it can generally be corrected. And you can choose from multiple methods of hormonal contraception to reduce your bleeding.

You don't have to live with pain during periods.

23

Period cramping comes from the chemicals released in your body. These chemicals cause uterine contractions that expel the uterine lining. This pain is real — not just an excuse to get out of gym class or to avoid a party with people you don't like. Having endometriosis or uterine fibroids can make this cramping even worse. And as many as 1 in 3 people with periods have pain (severe dysmenorrhea) bad enough that it interferes with daily activities. It can cause anxiety, make it hard to think straight, and even cause nausea and vomiting.

Though cramps with periods may be considered normal, you don't have to tough them out. Try a heating pad or hot shower or soak — heat can be your best friend. Avoid caffeine during your period — it can make cramping worse. Try ibuprofen and naproxen — you can get them at the drugstore or grocery store. If the recommended doses of these drugs aren't enough, ask your doctor for prescriptions for a higher dose. Almost all forms of hormonal contraception can take away pain, too. Taking any of these meds won't stop your uterus from contracting as much as it needs to. (In other words, bleeding won't build up in your uterus.)

24 You don't have to live with PMS.

Premenstrual syndrome (PMS) is a combination of symptoms that start right before or during your period and can be physical (fatigue, breast tenderness, bloating) or emotional (irritability, anxiety, sadness). Over 90% of women in the U.S. experience at least one symptom of PMS around their periods. And around 20% to 30% of women will experience multiple symptoms.

For some people, PMS is mild or occasional. But others have to miss school or work because their symptoms are so severe. Then there's the 3% to 8% of women who experience the most debilitating form, premenstrual dysphoric disorder (PMDD). PMDD can cause sudden and extreme mood swings, irritability, anger, depression and hopelessness.

You're not imagining or exaggerating these feelings — they're caused by huge hormonal swings. In the days before your bleeding begins, estrogen levels nose-dive. (Estrogen is linked to serotonin, a natural mood-regulating hormone.) Around the same time, your progesterone levels spike before they, too, drop. (Progesterone is a hormone that's linked to anxiety and depression for some people.)

Prescription medication, like birth control, antidepressants and anti-anxiety medications, can offer relief. Want to avoid meds? Practice self-care throughout the month. Get enough sleep and exercise, eat healthy, avoid smoking and excessive alcohol use, and use your best strategies for coping with stress.

Listen to your gut (and your uterus).

25

Sometimes you may feel like things aren't quite right with your periods — and period changes can be a sign of something larger going on with your health. Periods that have become heavy may mean you have uterine fibroids or thyroid disease. Spotting, especially after sex, may mean you have a polyp or a sexually transmitted infection. And terrible pain with your periods may signify endometriosis. You know your body better than anyone.

The best thing you can do if you feel like something's not right is to keep a period diary.

Don't let yourself fall down the internet rabbit hole of trying to figure out what's going on. Track your symptoms and rate how bad they are (try using a scale of 1 to 10) and when they come. This data can help make your case when you talk to your gyno or primary care doctor. But some doctors don't heed a person's concerns the first time they're raised. For instance, on average, a person can have symptoms for five to 10 years before getting diagnosed with endometriosis. So keep talking until someone takes your concerns seriously. This means that your doctor explains why if there's nothing to worry about, and lets you know what signs are cause for concern.

Period Checkup

Assess your periods by tracking them for several months and answering these questions:

- ☐ How long are my cycles? Are they between 21 and 35 days?
- ☐ How predictable are my periods? Do they vary in length?
- ☐ How many products do I use each day? Do I ever bleed through my products?
- ☐ Do I ever skip my period? Am I skipping more than one or two periods a year?
- ☐ How long are my periods? Do they last between three and seven days?
- ☐ Am I spotting between my periods?
- ☐ Do I ever miss school, work, or activities due to pain with my periods?
- ☐ Are my PMS symptoms manageable, or are they getting in the way of my life?

Ask Your Doctor...

I encourage you to ask your doctor any of these questions:

☐ Are my periods typical?

☐ What kinds of experiences have your patients had with menstrual cups and period underwear?

☐ Can I use birth control to control my periods? How would that work?

☐ Can we talk about ways to make my periods lighter?

☐ What can I do to make my cramping better?

☐ I feel awful with my period every month. What treatment do you recommend?

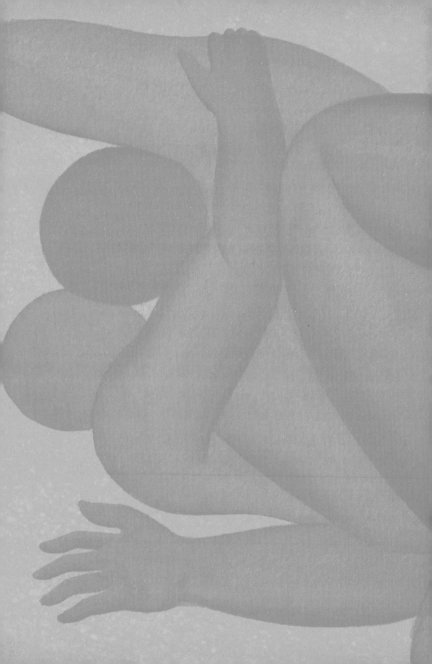

Desire, dryness and dildos

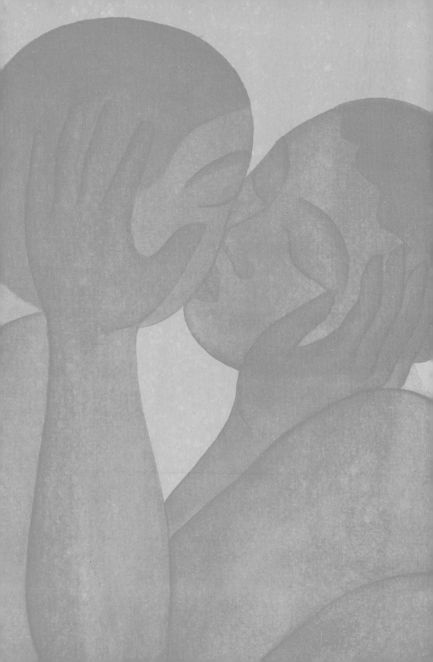

26. Masturbation is a wonderful teacher.

27. Your first time may not be what you expect.

28. A partner who doesn't have a clitoris may not know where yours is.

29. You may need more foreplay than you're getting.

30. Keep a bottle of lubricant at the bedside.

31. Sex shouldn't hurt.

32. No glove, no love.

33. Orgasms don't often come from intercourse alone.

34. It doesn't matter how you get an orgasm.

35. It's not all about the orgasm.

36. Take care of your toys.

37. Treat anal intercourse differently than P-in-V sex.

38. It's OK if you want more sex than others do.

39. It's OK if you don't want sex as much as others do.

40. It's OK if you don't want sex *at all*.

41. Consent is only the beginning.

42. You can get an STI from sex that isn't P-in-V.

43. Even if you trust your partner, let me test you for STIs.

26 Masturbation is a wonderful teacher.

Your first sexual experience may be with yourself — and that's a fantastic introduction to sex and pleasure. There's no issue with consent, no risk of infection or pregnancy, and no one to please but yourself. Another reason masturbation is so important? You learn about your body. Through touching yourself, you can learn what kind of touch turns you on — firm or soft, circles or pulses, flicking or tapping, and up-and-down or side-to-side motions. And you get to explore *where* you like to be touched. Almost any area of the body can be an erogenous zone with the right contact, in the right situation.

When you're with yourself, no touching is off-limits. (But stick to using your fingers and objects designed for this purpose.) You may prefer to be alone, and locked doors can be a comfort. Know that masturbation is completely healthy. If you listen to your body, you're not going to hurt yourself or spoil yourself for partnered sex.

A bedtime orgasm can be a fabulous sleep aid.

Touching yourself can even boost your body image and raise your self-esteem. And once you know what feels good, you can let future partners know, making partnered sex all the better.

Your first time may not be what you expect.

27

Rarely is your first time having sex with a partner like what you've seen in a movie, on TV, or in porn. No one is that smooth or that sure of themselves. And someone is going to bump someone else with their head or elbow at some point. It's OK to be nervous, to not be aroused or lubricated enough (more on that next). It's also OK to *not* be nervous and to be thrilled to be having sex with a person you like.

With a little thinking in advance, you can help make your first time one that you'll remember with a grin. Make sure sex with this person at this moment is what you want. Get enough foreplay that your whole body is ready for the next step. If you're well-versed in how your body responds to different kinds of touch (thanks, masturbation!), let your partner know. Seriously consider using a condom if your partner has a penis so you're not left with an STI as a parting gift. And don't rush it — make sure you have enough time both before and after to connect with your partner.

28 A partner who doesn't have a clitoris may not know where yours is.

Sex education classes don't teach teens *nearly* enough about anatomy and sex. When my stepson was a sophomore, I peppered him with questions about what he learned in school. I was horrified by how limited the coverage was, and sometimes what he learned was just plain wrong. As a gyno, I feel like there should be an entire semester devoted to these things. Most peoples' parents don't teach their kids about sex and the body. It's hard for the people who changed your diapers to think about you as a sexual being.

When sex ed happens in schools, boys and girls generally learn in separate classrooms, so it's common for boys to not know anything about the female body. They don't understand periods, may be mystified by anatomy, and may not know that you have three holes (urethra, vagina and anus) — yup, it's true, you don't pee out of your vagina.

In addition, your partner may not know what makes you feel good. So, you'll need to speak up about how you want your body touched. Do you want your breasts handled firmly, caressed, or left alone? Is your bum an erogenous zone for you? And make sure your partner knows that a clitoris needs to be treated more gently than a penis does.

You may need more foreplay than you're getting.

29

When both your body and your brain are aroused, sex is more comfortable and fun, even when it doesn't involve something inside of you. When you get aroused, the blood vessels in the pelvis widen (dilate). This rush of blood southward swells (engorges) the vulva, and the vagina expands and deepens. This increased blood flow to the vagina also causes fluid to pass through the walls. That's the main source of what makes you feel wet (lubricated). All this bodily magic takes time.

> **The best sex comes when you have both mental (between your ears) and physical (between your legs) arousal.**

How you're feeling emotionally is even more important than how your vagina is responding. And it may take some time before your brain catches up with your body.

Know that you're not being high-maintenance for needing more than a few minutes of foreplay. This isn't to say that quickies are dangerous, and some people do get aroused in a flash (lucky ducks). But it's completely OK to ask for what you need. Remember that the better sex feels for you, the more you're going to want to have it, and everybody wins.

30 Keep a bottle of lubricant at the bedside.

Even if your partner gets you fully turned on, you may find that your natural moisture isn't enough to make intercourse comfortable. Everyone makes different amounts of moisture, and being wet doesn't always mean you're aroused (and vice versa). Plus, it's common to start feeling dry if intercourse lasts awhile. Adding lube — on the penis and at the vaginal or internal genital opening — can make penetration much more comfortable.

And lube improves more than P-in-V sex. For anal sex, lube is needed to reduce the risk of injury. It's also great for hand jobs. You may even want to use lube when you masturbate, for a different sensation.

You can get lube at the grocery store, pharmacy or online. The right one lasts as long as you need it to and doesn't irritate you during or after sex. Try a water-based lube to start. Silicone-based ones are OK if you're not also using toys made of silicone. If you want to use a silicone lube with silicone toys, do a patch test on the toy first to make sure they won't stick together.

Water-based and silicone lubes are both fine with condoms, but oil-based lubes will dissolve the latex in condoms. Warming lubes have chemicals that risk stinging and irritation, so you may be better off simply warming the lube in your hand before use.

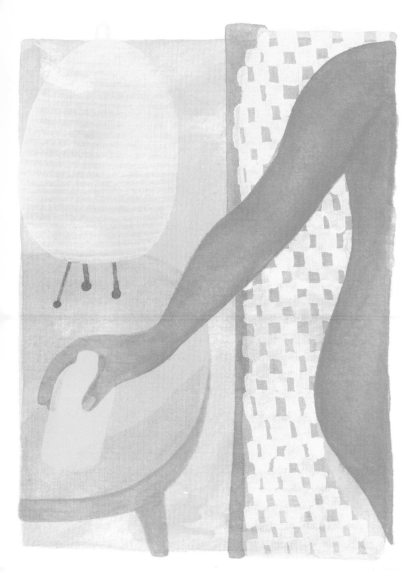

31 Sex shouldn't hurt.

Conversations and education often don't center on what vaginal intercourse should *feel* like, whether your partner has a penis or not. And if your first experience with intercourse wasn't comfortable, you may think that it's supposed to be like that.

But it's not. While sex may *sometimes* be uncomfortable if you're not fully aroused, **sex should not cause you pain**. Full stop.

Sadly, though, painful sex is common. As many as 1 in 5 women in the U.S. will experience pain with intercourse (dyspareunia). Sex may be especially uncomfortable if you haven't had penetrative sex in a while. But just because it's common, it doesn't mean you have to accept it. Pushing through the pain only reinforces the message to your body that pain comes from being touched. That's a tough feedback loop to break once it's been in place for a while.

If sex hurts, stop what you're doing. If more foreplay and adding lube don't do the trick, see your gyno, who can see what may be causing your pain. Sometimes pain is related to a recent pregnancy or your birth control method or may be caused by pain elsewhere, such as back pain or menstrual cramps. There are many things that can help you, including medications and pelvic floor physical therapy. Your doctor can help you find the right pain relief.

No glove, no love.

32

Condoms during intercourse offer peace of mind for two reasons. They'll reduce your risk of a sexually transmitted infection (STI), and they'll help protect against a pregnancy you're not ready for. Most condoms are made of latex, but some are made from polyurethane for those with a latex allergy. Avoid ones made of lambskin, as they won't protect you from STIs.

If you feel awkward asking your partner to wear a condom, I suggest following the 3 Rules of Rubbers:

1 Communicate, in your words and body language, that you *expect* your partner to wear a condom. In other words: You're not making a request! Don't pose it as a question.

2 Have condoms at the ready — so you can unwrap one at the right time — or ask if your partner has one to use. In other words: That's the only choice there is.

3 If your partner still doesn't want to wear one, brightly say that you're OK with play that doesn't involve bodily fluids. In other words: No glove, no love.

Setting an expectation that condoms will be used — and coming prepared with your own stash — is the best way to not feel bad about asking.

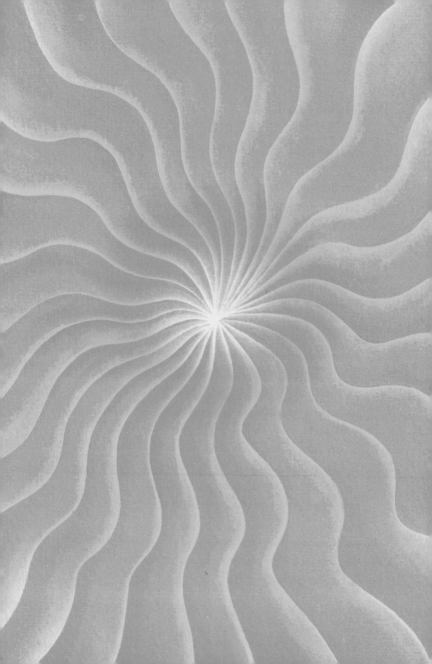

Orgasms don't often come from intercourse alone.

33

Fewer than 1 in 5 women say they can climax from vaginal intercourse alone — everyone else wants or needs some sort of stimulation on their clitoris. Your clit can be stimulated directly, but for some people that's too intense, and they prefer indirect stimulation, including from the side through the labia, with gentle pulling on the labia minora, or even through clothing. Touching in or around the vagina, including on the perineum and under the urethra, may stimulate the inner portion of the clitoris (which extends way beyond the nub you know and love, extending in the shape of a wishbone behind the vaginal wall into the pelvis). Check out MayoClinic.org and search on *vulva* to see how everything is connected.

If you want to try to have an orgasm during vaginal penetration, try stimulating your clitoris at the same time. Either touch yourself with your fingers or a vibrator or have your partner touch you. Aim for the area around your clitoris. If that feels too much like a game of Twister, try manual or oral stimulation before or after intercourse. Other kinds of touching during intercourse, including kissing, licking and sucking, can also help get you there.

34 It doesn't matter how you get an orgasm.

Even the most caring partner may not consistently push your buttons the right way. And it can be challenging to manage direct clitoral stimulation during intercourse, depending on how flexible you can be with your sex positions. If having orgasms with a partner doesn't come easy for you, try using a vibrator. Vibes come in many forms, and most are battery-operated so they can be moved about your body without cords getting in the way. With practice, you can get the hang of timing your climax for the moment that feels best for you.

A vibrator may be your ticket to timing your orgasms with your partner's, especially during intercourse.

Some patients make a face when I suggest introducing a vibrator into their couple's time. They've always seen a vibe as something for private, personal play. But there's nothing wrong with a battery-operated assist to get you over the edge. For partners who seem hesitant — as if they're being left out of the game — let them wield the wand. It may take practice and communication to get the angle, intensity and pacing right. But what a lovely thing to practice.

It's not all about the orgasm.

35

You can get a lot out of simply being close with someone: Connecting after a hard day at work or in a time of grief. Satisfying "skin hunger" and the need to be touched and held. Enjoying sexual playtime and trying new things. And maybe feeling the satisfaction and joy of giving your partner an orgasm. Great sex doesn't mean everyone climaxes — great sex happens when everyone feels good and wants to do it again.

Whether you have an orgasm or not, sex also has a lot of surprising health benefits. Sex can lower your blood pressure and improve your heart health. It can strengthen your immune system and decrease symptoms of depression and anxiety. Sex can lead to better sleep, pain relief, and stress reduction, both physical and emotional. A healthy sex life may even improve your self-esteem and boost your libido, so you want more of a good thing! You get these benefits with or without an orgasm.

36 Take care of your toys.

After a satisfying sex session, you may be tempted to roll over and pass out. But in the name of good health, do these before you snooze: Brush your teeth and floss. Pee, so you flush out any bacteria. Replace your birth control ring or menstrual cup if you removed it for sex. And take care of any toys you may have used during the fun.

Clean any toy that was exposed to bodily fluids, even if it never entered a body cavity. Just use soap and water. A washcloth can get into the crevices of a toy with nubs, such as a vibrator. There are also sex toy cleansing wipes, perfect if you don't have access to running water. Take out the batteries if the toy is going to be left unused for a while — it's sad to find an exploded battery in a vibe that you pull out months after its last use. Tuck all your toys out of the reach of dogs and children. The former because you don't want Peppa the Pug to mistake your dildo for a chew toy. And the latter not because you shouldn't talk about sex, but because you might not be ready to explain it, or simply want to keep your private life private.

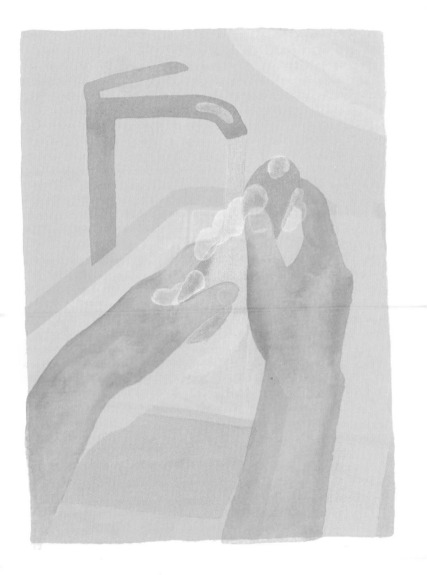

37 Treat anal intercourse differently than P-in-V sex.

Anal sex isn't just backdoor intercourse. It's the insertion of fingers, toys or anything else into the bum for sexual pleasure. And it's fairly common: One U.S. survey shows that 36% of women and 42% of men have had anal sex.

Want to try backdoor play? Five rules to keep it safe and fun:

1 **Use *plenty* of water-based lube.** The anus and rectum can't self-lubricate like the vagina does.
2 **Allow time to relax the muscle** (anal sphincter) before anything enters you. The anus and rectum have a thinner lining than that of the vagina or mouth, so they need to be treated more gingerly.
3 **Have your partner rock back and forth** instead of thrusting in and out. The rectum wasn't built to withstand piston-like thrusting, like what you may have with vaginal sex. Having vigorous anal sex risks small tears in your anus or rectum.
4 ***Always* use a condom without spermicide.** Those tears may not bleed and may be too small to see. However, they increase your risk of acquiring HIV and other sexually transmitted diseases.
5 **If you have any pain, stop.** This is the most important rule of all.

It's OK if you want more sex than others do.

38

If you identify as a woman, you may be treated negatively for enjoying sex or even just having it. But being sexual is part of what makes us human, so you shouldn't be judged for wanting any amount of sex that feels right (and oh-so-good).

There is no "normal" amount of sex to want or have. And lesbian and bisexual women report having as much sex as hetero women each year. Yet people's expectations about how much sex they *think* you should want or have are shaped by society, culture and religion. If you're with a male partner, he may have been taught to be the sexual aggressor and be used to setting the sexual pace. As a result, he may react badly when you show that you want to set the tempo, especially if it's faster than he would set it. Or your partner's libido, regardless of gender, may simply be lower than yours.

No matter the reason for the imbalance, it's OK if you want sex more than your partner does. Don't let any partner shame you for your desires. You'll have to figure out how to negotiate this gap, but that should come from a healthy place, not one of judgment.

39 It's OK if you don't want sex as much as others do.

There's no gold standard in terms of how much sex you should want or have. It's OK if you run at a lower RPM (romps per month) than your partner does or than your friends do. And it's common to have a lower sex drive with stress, illness, pain, fear of pregnancy, or fear of getting caught — and then rebound when those things pass. The reality is that about half of women have sex at least once a week — everyone else is having sex less often. And there's also no rule about what *kind* of sex to want, either. You may love oral sex because it reliably gets you off and feel meh about intercourse. Or the opposite — maybe intercourse makes you feel connected to your partner and oral is too intense.

Either way, you may find yourself with a sexual mismatch with your partner. But it doesn't mean there's something wrong with you. There's nothing wrong with not wanting sex as much as your partner does, or your friends do. If you're unhappy with how disinterested you are in sex, talk with your doctor. But if you're content with the amount of sex you're wanting, you're OK. You deserve to be with a partner who travels at the same sexual speed as you, and who won't make you feel pressured to have sex when you don't want to.

It's OK if you don't want sex *at all*.

40

Many people (and doctors) assume that all people want and experience sexual desire and attraction. But not everyone experiences sexual attraction to others. People who don't experience consistent sexual attraction often consider themselves asexual, or ace.

There's a wide spectrum of feelings within the asexual label. Aces may sometimes feel attraction and may even fall in love. Or may be attracted to people but not desire sex with them. Attraction to others may be only occasional (graysexual) or only after forming a deep, emotional connection with a partner (demisexual). It's important to know that each ace experiences attraction and relationships in unique ways. And then there's the relationship between sex and romance. Aromantic people may experience sexual attraction, but not have a rom-com attraction to a partner.

Asexuality is a label for sexual *attraction*, not sex drive or arousal or enjoyment with sex. So, it's common for aces to masturbate, have a high libido, or even have fun during sex in certain circumstances. If you've ever wondered why you don't seem to feel the same way as your friends when it comes to sex and relationships, the *aces* world may be the right fit.

41 Consent is only the beginning. Trigger warning: unwanted sexual activity.

Consent is the very least you should have with your partner — for everything from touching your body to intercourse of any variety. Some people mock the idea of "affirmative sex" and getting permission for every kiss and touch. But the only way you know if your partner is as into your play as much as you are, is to check in as things progress. It doesn't have to always be a verbal question. A raised eyebrow and then waiting for something in return (a "yes," a nod, maybe a moan) may be enough. The goal is for both of you to have the space to signal when things should slow down or stop fully.

> **Everyone has the right to revoke consent at any point in play for any reason.**

Another approach you may explore is to give your partner the opportunity to light your fire even if it's not lit at the start. This is called being persuadable. People tend to think that sexual arousal proceeds in a straight line — first you experience desire, then you get aroused, then (if you're lucky) you have an orgasm. But people can experience sexual response in multiple ways, and it's shaped like a circle more than a line. Desire may come *after* arousal, and the two may enhance each other. This means that sometimes getting playful and intimate with a partner will trigger desire, even if you don't feel it at the start. And we know that external factors — such as how close you feel to a person, the dynamic of your relationship, and what sex means for you in this moment — all contribute to your sexual response.

And know there's a difference between sex you consent to and sex you want. It's totally possible to consent to unwanted sex. You may agree to sex only to please your partner, or to avoid tension or a fight. You may feel obligated to have sex after a date (even though you shouldn't) or feel that you don't want to disappoint your partner. Or you may be afraid of your partner losing interest or breaking up with you. Unwanted yet consensual sex can happen in a number of situations, regardless of the gender or sexuality of the partners, or the seriousness of the relationship.

You may need to sit with the idea of this for a while. It's OK if you feel OK about these encounters — you have agency over your body, and I want you to feel that you can make what feel like the right decisions for you. But you may not be feeling OK about what has happened. If you're feeling traumatized by anything sexually that has happened in your past, please talk to your doctor.

42 You can get an STI from sex that isn't P-in-V.

When people think about sex that puts them at risk for sexually transmitted infections, they tend to think about penile-vaginal intercourse. It's true that penetrative sex, especially receptive anal sex, is the highest risk for HIV transmission. But P-in-V sex isn't the only kind of activity that runs a risk of STIs. You can get oral STIs from going down on your partner. You can get STIs from anal intercourse, whether you're giving or receiving. And women who don't identify as straight aren't any less at risk than heterosexual women, even though many think they're so safe that they don't get vaccinated or screened regularly. HPV and herpes are the trickiest of all, as they only need skin-to-skin contact with an infected person. HPV can even be transmitted through mutual masturbation or sharing unclean sex toys.

So, everyone needs to think about reducing their infection risk when having partnered sex. That means going beyond just condoms on penises. Put condoms on your sex toys, use finger cots for all kinds of penetration, and whip out the dental dams when going down. And let your gyno know what kinds of sex you have, so they know where to swab you.

Even if you trust your partner, let me test you for STIs.

Not all people regularly use condoms when having penile-vaginal intercourse. Many people enjoy intercourse more when they're not using condoms. Some partners think a request to use condoms is a sign that you're having sex with other people. And you may be a condom-user on the reg, but sometimes you're having such a good time that you simply don't want to stop the fun to put one on. I understand all these reasons…but STIs don't care.

I often hear from my patients that they're in a relationship in which they don't feel like they're at risk of an STI and they don't need to use condoms. But I've diagnosed chlamydia in way too many people (including a 50-something-year-old grandmother) to believe that everyone is as safe from STIs as they feel. These infections are often silent until they wreak havoc with your fertility or cause chronic pelvic pain. So, consider a "trust but verify" approach to STI screening. Annual testing is easy, just a simple swab and blood tests. If you want, you can tell your partner it's just routine. And ideally, your partner will also get tested, and you can swap your results before you swap fluids.

Sex Checkup

Many of my patients wonder if they're typical or healthy. Ask yourself these questions — and then talk with your gyno if you're not happy with your answers.

- ☐ Am I getting enough foreplay before any penetrative sex?
- ☐ Am I having any pain with sex?
- ☐ Do I have any trouble getting aroused?
- ☐ Do I have any issues with orgasm?
- ☐ Am I happy with how much sex I'm wanting?
- ☐ Am I happy with how much sex I'm having?
- ☐ Have I consented to unwanted sex? How do I feel about that?
- ☐ Do I need to get intoxicated to have sex?
- ☐ Do I feel safe in my relationship?
- ☐ Am I using condoms or latex barriers whenever I want to?

Ask Your Doctor...

I encourage you to ask your doctor any of these questions:

☐ I've never masturbated before. Do you have any advice?

☐ I've never had an orgasm before. Do you have any advice?

☐ What kinds of lubricant do you recommend?

☐ Why does it hurt when I try to have intercourse or use a tampon?

☐ How can I try anal sex in a safe way?

☐ What STIs can you test me for?

☐ I don't want sex as much as I used to, and it's bothering me. How can I boost my sex drive?

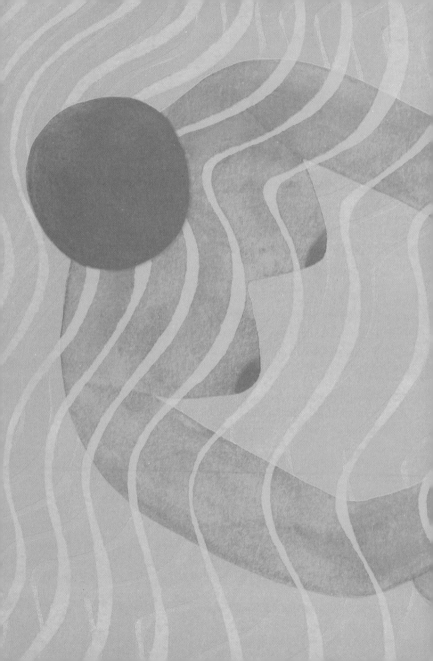

How to plan your fam

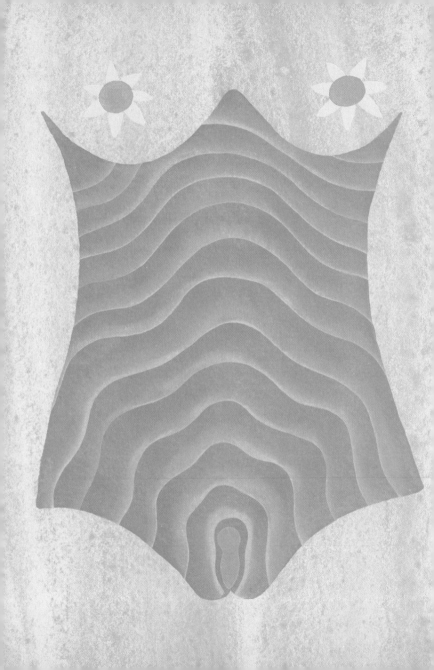

44. If you have eggs and your partner has sperm, think about contraception.

45. If you've never gotten pregnant, it doesn't mean you can't get pregnant.

46. You should only use contraception if you want to.

47. The pill protects you from more than pregnancy.

48. The pill isn't your only birth control option.

49. The 'morning-after pill' is good for 5 mornings-after.

50. Pulling out is not pointless.

51. All birth control is safer than pregnancy.

52. Even abortion is safer than pregnancy.

53. You can use more than one method of birth control.

54. You get to control your contraception.

55. Birth control won't hurt your fertility.

56. Abortion won't hurt your fertility.

44 If you have eggs and your partner has sperm, think about contraception.

Pregnancy isn't related to identity or orientation — it's related to your organs and your sex cells. No matter your gender identity or sexual orientation, if you have at least one functioning ovary and fallopian tube, and your partner has sperm that is deposited near your cervix, you have a chance of becoming pregnant. That may be what you want — or it may be anything but.

If it's the latter, talk to your doctor about all your contraceptive options. You may want a method that works all the time and that you don't have to think about. At my hospital, we frequently place intrauterine devices (IUDs) in patients either in the office or under sedation at their request — especially helpful for some trans and nonbinary folks. Or you may prefer a method that you only use when you're going to have sex that involves sperm. If you're taking testosterone, you have multiple choices for birth control that won't interfere with T or your transition.

If you're a trans man, taking testosterone is not reliable birth control, but you can use any contraceptive method, even the hormonal ones.

If you've never gotten pregnant, it doesn't mean you can't get pregnant.

45

I've had many patients shocked by a positive pregnancy test. Maybe they hadn't used contraception for years and had never been pregnant. Or their partner believed they couldn't parent a child, and therefore they didn't need birth control. Maybe they're managing a illness that makes their periods irregular.

Pregnancy is mysterious. Some people try for pregnancy for years, without success. Others conceive the very first time they have P-in-V sex. Patients with polycystic ovarian syndrome or endometriosis may struggle to get pregnant when they want, but then have an out-of-the-blue pregnancy. If you have at least one ovary, at least one tube, a uterus, and a sperm-producing partner, you may be able to get pregnant.

When medical professionals say you *can't* get pregnant, they often don't mean that you are unable to. What they're often trying to say is that you *shouldn't* get pregnant.

You're also almost never too sick to become pregnant. If you're managing a chronic illness and desperately want to get pregnant, work with your care team to get in the best possible health before you conceive. And if pregnancy isn't recommended by your doctors — especially if it could hurt or even kill you — talk to your doctor about birth control.

46 You should only use contraception if you want to.

The decision to use birth control — or not — is an intensely personal one. Plenty of people don't think about pregnancy as something you *plan*, but as something that happens when it's meant to. Others have a "whatever happens, happens" philosophy and don't want to take any actions to stop a pregnancy from occurring. And plenty of people have experienced the fact that no matter how well you plan, sometimes pregnancy is out of your hands. I have patients who've gotten pregnant multiple times despite perfect use of different kinds of birth control, and others who can't get pregnant no matter how hard they try.

A lot of factors are at play when you're deciding whether to use birth control. Cost, privacy, side effects, period wackiness, how hard it is to get to a doctor's office…it's understandable why you may not want to worry about it. And if getting pregnant wouldn't be devastating for you, contraception may not feel like a high priority.

You also may have strong feelings about pregnancy that don't fit nicely into the usual "I use birth control because I'm not ready to get pregnant" or the "I'm not using birth control because I'm trying for a baby" lanes. It's OK to be unsure how you feel about getting pregnant, but you don't want to shut the door to the possibility, so don't want a device that stays inside your body. It's OK to not want to use a method that your doctor thinks is the best thing ever, or more effective than the one you've chosen. It's OK to want to get pregnant even when other people think you shouldn't. These feelings often drive your decision to use a particular method of contraception, or no contraception at all. Be open with your partner about your feelings about birth control, and what you want to use (or not use). But it's no one else's business what you decide. Don't let anyone — your partner, your family, or your health care provider — talk you into using contraception if it doesn't feel right to you.

47 The pill protects you from more than pregnancy.

There are so many benefits from the birth control pill that I think it should be called the better-quality-of-life pill.

Using the combination birth control pill leads to shorter, predictable periods that may last only a few days. (When I was using the pill, my period would always start on a Tuesday and last precisely four days.) Your flow is lighter on pills, too — some people need to use pads or tampons for only a day or two, and then switch to liners. Most people have less cramping, which is particularly awesome if you have endometriosis. You'll have fewer ovarian cysts. You're at less risk of anemia, which is when you don't have enough healthy red blood cells to get the oxygen your body needs where it needs to go.

Using the pill for 10 or more years in your life lowers your chance of ovarian and uterine cancer by up to 50%.

You likely get these same benefits from other combined hormonal contraception methods, if using a weekly patch or the vaginal ring is more your speed.

The pill isn't your only birth control option.

48

Sometimes you have a love match with your birth control method. Your life feels better with it, you give glowing reviews to your friends, and you wonder why it took you so long to find it.

But sometimes it's a toxic relationship. It makes you miserable and maybe even causes you to hate your body. You may need to try multiple methods before you find the right one. And different methods may be right for different times in your life. There's absolutely no shame in having used multiple methods — I call it the birth control journey.

Switching your birth control method is very common and completely fine.

Take the pill, for example. It's a great method for many people, but it can be hard to take a pill every day. If you want light, predictable periods, there's a weekly patch and a monthly ring. If you want a "set it and forget it" method, there's an implant and several IUDs. Some methods you use with sex don't need a prescription, like spermicides and pulling out. If you want to go totally natural, you can track your body signs and use a fertility awareness method. Your doctor can help you figure out the best birth control for you.

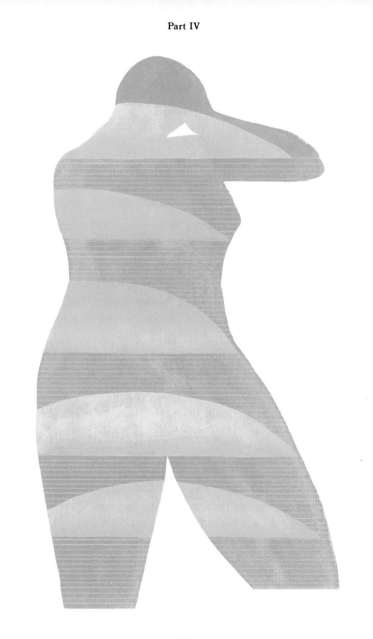

The 'morning-after pill' is good for 5 mornings-after.

49

Emergency contraception (EC) is birth control that you use after sex to prevent a pregnancy. EC is commonly known as the morning-after pill, but it's effective for up to 120 hours after sex. If the condom broke or you messed up another contraceptive method, get yourself a dose as soon as possible. And no, EC is not the same as the abortion pill — it won't interfere with a pregnancy that has already begun. EC is especially great to have on hand if you rarely have sex with a partner with a penis and don't need birth control all the time.

The most famous form of EC is Plan B One-Step, available at most pharmacies without a prescription. Plan B has generic forms that are just as effective — you can even order them online for as little as $15. If cost is a factor, many insurance plans cover Plan B, so ask your gyno for a prescription. The other pill form of EC is called ella. This one is more effective than Plan B four or five days after sex, so if you'll be taking EC a few days after sex, ella is the better choice.

Have a dose of EC already on hand for that unexpectedly good date or birth control breakdown.

A little-known fact is that EC pills lose their effectiveness if you have a higher body mass index (BMI). If your BMI is over 26 — if, for example, you're over 147 pounds and 5′3″ or over 166 pounds and 5′7″ — Plan B likely won't work for you. You can check your BMI using an app or online calculator. Ella is at least as effective, if not more effective, than Plan B for everyone who takes it. But ella is a bit weight-sensitive, too, and starts to lose its efficacy at a BMI of 35, which is over 198 pounds if you're 5′3″, or over 224 pounds if you're 5′7″.

The most effective EC of all is not a pill. An intrauterine device (IUD) is a T-shaped device that's inserted into your uterus by a doctor and can stay in your uterus for up to 10 years, depending on the model. Two kinds of IUD will work for EC: the copper IUD (Paragard) or the 52-mg levonorgestrel IUD (Mirena or Liletta). Both IUDs are 99% effective at preventing pregnancy, and they both work well no matter your weight.

The IUD can either be left in to provide ongoing birth control, or you can have it removed at the time of your next period. Once you know you need EC, get to your gyno ASAP.

Pulling out is not pointless.

50

Withdrawal, or pulling out, is free and easy to access, with no prescription or late-night trips to the pharmacy required. It's one of only three methods of contraception that people with a penis have control over (the others being external condoms and vasectomy). It's especially good if there's no other method of birth control available and you decide to have sex anyway. When used perfectly, it has only a 4% failure rate.

Withdrawal can be difficult to use perfectly, especially if your partner is inexperienced or intoxicated. And some people with penises can have sperm in their pre-cum (the fluid that comes out before ejaculation). Studies have shown that a person with a penis will tend to have sperm in the pre-cum, or they won't. Unfortunately, there's no easy way to know if your partner is a "leaker" or not. Because of both these reasons, the typical use failure rate for withdrawal is around 1 in 5.

Pulling out may be the right method for you some-times, or all the time. While you may want to choose a more effective method if pregnancy would be devastating, many people rely on withdrawal at least from time to time.

51 All birth control is safer than pregnancy.

Contraception needs a better publicist, because it gets horribly bad press whenever a person using it has a serious problem. It's easy to find websites and social media posts that make it seem like the risks are incredibly high — including some that are clearly trying to scare people into not using birth control at all. Many people have an inner skepticism of using birth control that contains hormones. They feel that artificial hormones aren't natural and may even be dangerous.

Thankfully, there's more than 60 years' worth of research on the hormones used in contraception, both the estrogen component (usually ethinyl estradiol) and the progesterone one (varieties of progestin). And these mountains of research are all consistent about the overall safety of hormones. The most significant risk of using estrogen is developing a blood clot in a leg or lung, but that risk and others are incredibly low for healthy people. Your doctor will screen you for the health conditions that make using hormonal birth control risky.

Birth control hormones aren't harmful.

However, what the media rarely addresses is the risks of *pregnancy* — which far outweigh the risks of birth control. No one gives these risks a lot of thought because doctors don't stress to pregnant people just how dangerous pregnancy can be. When you start getting prenatal care, your obstetrician doesn't make you sign a consent form acknowledging all the risks. If pregnancy required a long package insert like birth control does, it would tell you that the risks of pregnancy include high blood pressure (preeclampsia), diabetes, blood clots, stroke, hemorrhage/transfusion, hysterectomy, and even death.

If you're having sex that puts you at risk of pregnancy and you don't want to be pregnant, using birth control is the safest way to go. Talk with your doctor about your medical history, and he or she will discuss all the risks and benefits of each method of contraception you're interested in. Together you can find a method of contraception that doesn't make you worry and may even improve your quality of life.

52 Even abortion is safer than pregnancy.

Based on how abortion is depicted on TV and in movies, you'd think you're taking your life in your hands by having one. But what you see on screen is an unrealistic portrayal. In truth, most people are completely fine physically *and* emotionally. The rate of complications with a first-trimester abortion, most of them not serious, is less than 1%. The most common emotion people have after an abortion is relief, and you're back to work or school in three days — but that doesn't make for much of a dramatic story.

You might be surprised to learn that the riskiest thing a pregnant person can do is to stay pregnant. But carrying a baby to term carries far greater risks to your health than an abortion does. In fact, carrying a pregnancy to term is 14 times more likely to kill you than having an abortion — a risk that's higher for Black and Latinx people than white. And if you have serious medical problems that make a pregnancy life-threatening, abortion is even safer.

Of course, safety alone is generally not the reason to choose an abortion. If you're getting good prenatal care, you're likely to come through pregnancy unscathed. But if you find yourself in the position of needing an abortion, know that you're not doing something dangerous for your body by terminating the pregnancy.

You can use more than one method of birth control.

53

You may look at a poster in your doctor's office of all the available contraceptive methods and think, "How do I pick just one?" Happily, you don't have to.

There are three reasons you might want to use two methods of birth control at one time:

- Effectiveness may be very important to you, but you may not want to use an IUD or an implant (the methods with the highest efficacy). In this case, you can "double up" your birth control to make your contraceptive plan more effective. Think using the pill and pulling out, or condoms and spermicide.
- You may want to have STI protection in addition to contraception and want a stronger or more effective plan than using condoms alone. If your partner with a penis doesn't want to wear a condom and you're willing to have sex anyway, think about Phexxi, the vaginal gel. It can help protect you from chlamydia and gonorrhea infection (but not from HIV or other viruses).
- You may want one method of birth control for its high effectiveness and another to treat a separate problem. For example, you may use a copper IUD and the pill to improve your acne.

54 You get to control your contraception.

When you know you want to stop or switch contraception, you often want to do it ASAP. With most methods, your fertility returns to baseline as soon as you stop using it. So, if you're not ready for a pregnancy yet, you may want to start using something else right away, such as condoms or pulling out, until you choose another method. It can be tricky to get a follow-up appointment with your doctor to talk about birth control, so see if you can get a telemedicine visit sooner.

But there are doctors who may encourage you to try a method a little longer. They may say things like, "Your body needs time to get used to it." Or "Those side effects aren't serious." Or even, "You haven't had the device in that long, so it's a waste to take it out." These doctors may mean well, not wanting you to have a pregnancy that they think you don't want. But regardless of their intentions, they don't know what's best for you when it comes to your contraception.

It's your body and you don't need to leave anything on it or inside it if you don't want to. Want to stop the pill after using it for three months? Just stop.

Don't throw away that abandoned half-used pill pack — those leftover pills may be useful as emergency contraception someday. (Ask your gyno how to do it.)

Want the IUD out at your six-week post-insertion string check? Be clear with your gyno that you're not leaving the office with the IUD still in place. And if the thought of arguing with your doctor makes your stomach churn, it may be a sign that it's time for a new doctor. Every health care provider should trust that you know what's best for you and for your life, and that includes what you do about contraception.

55 Birth control won't hurt your fertility.

When contraception works well for a very long time, it's natural to wonder, *Can I still get pregnant?* Many (but not all) birth control users want their fertility to come back some day. And even more people don't like the idea of using something for contraception that could hurt their pregnancy options in the future.

The great news is that contraception will *not* reduce your fertility. All the hormonal methods are immediately reversible except for the injection, which can delay your next ovulation by a year. No method has a permanent effect on your ovaries, your tubes or the lining of your uterus. So, when you stop using birth control, your fertility returns to what it would have been if you'd never used it.

Sterilization, though, is forever. When you have part or all of your fallopian tubes removed, that's it. There's no "untying" your tubes, and there's no such thing as a five-year tubal ligation. Once you're *absolutely sure* you don't want to get pregnant, sterilization can be a great option.

You're (almost) never too young or too old to be sterilized, if this is truly what you want.

Abortion won't hurt your fertility.

56

I have people in my office struggling to get pregnant, wondering if the abortion they had when they were younger is the reason why they can't get pregnant now. Even some patients who are having a miscarriage wonder if their long-ago abortion is the reason.

I promise you, having an uncomplicated abortion will not harm your ability to get pregnant in the future. It won't scar your uterus or damage your cervix. In fact, you can get pregnant in as little as 8 to 10 days after a first-trimester abortion. That's how quickly your fertility returns.

Why do I say "uncomplicated"? It's natural to fear complications with any medical procedure. Even the most common abortion complication — needing an additional procedure — happens to fewer than 3% of people, with no lasting damage to your body. The chance of having a problem during an abortion that prevents you from having future pregnancies is less than the chance of being struck by lightning. It's also much less than the chance of losing your uterus (hysterectomy) from a pregnancy complication.

Birth Control Checkup

The best way to talk to your doctor about birth control is to know what's important to you. What do you want your contraception to do for you? Use this guide to sort it out.

☐ Do you want to see bleeding every month?
  → Think about the pill, patch, ring and the copper IUD.

☐ Do you *not* want to see bleeding every month?
  → Think about continuous pill or ring use, the injection or the 52-mg hormonal IUDs.

☐ Are you OK with spotting in between your periods, or would that be a nightmare?
  → To avoid the potential of long-term spotting, avoid progestin-only pills, the 19.5- and 52-mg hormonal IUDs, and the implant.

☐ Do you need a method to reduce your menstrual cramps or your acne?
  → Your best friend may be a pill, patch or ring.

☐ Do you need to keep your birth control private?
  → Consider the injection, implant or IUDs.

☐ Do you want one of the most effective methods?
  → Your best bets are the IUDs and the implant.

☐ Do you want a method that you only have to use when you're having sex with a sperm-producing partner?

→ Stock up on condoms, spermicide, Phexxi or a diaphragm/cervical cap.

☐ Do you want a method where you can "set it and forget it"?

→ You get months-long use with the injection and continuous use of the one-year ring and years-long use with the IUDs and implant.

☐ Do you want a method that can also protect you from sexually transmitted infections?

→ Condoms are the most reliable for preventing all STIs, while Phexxi can protect against chlamydia and gonorrhea.

☐ Is it OK if a method goes on or inside your body?

→ If not, avoid the patch, ring, IUDs and implants.

☐ Do you want to be able to stop and start the method without needing a doctor?

→ If so, avoid the implant and the IUD (though you can remove the IUD yourself!).

☐ Do you want your fertility to come back immediately when you stop using it?

→ All methods are green-lit except for the injection.

Ask Your Doctor...

I encourage you to ask your doctor any of these questions:

☐ Does anything in my medical history mean I shouldn't use certain birth control methods?

☐ Can you give me a prescription for a year's worth of pills/patches/rings, so I don't have to go to the pharmacy every month?

☐ Can I have a prescription for emergency contraception?

☐ I've had awful experiences with hormonal methods in the past. What birth control without hormones can you recommend for me?

☐ I love the idea of an IUD, but I'm scared of the insertion. Can I get sedation for the procedure?

☐ I never want to have (or have more) children. Can you talk with me about tubal ligation?

☐ If I need an abortion, can I see you for it or would you refer me to another doctor?

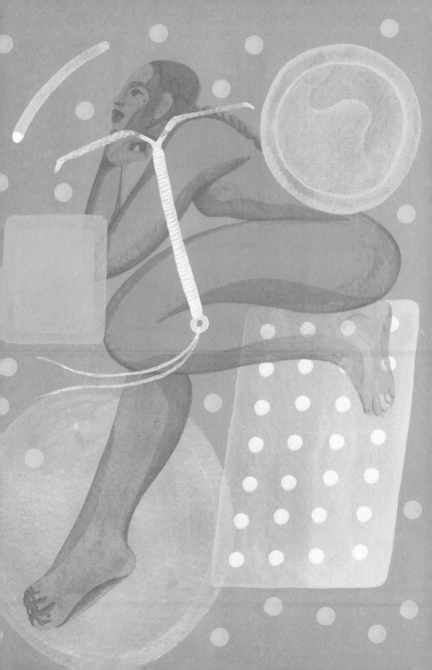

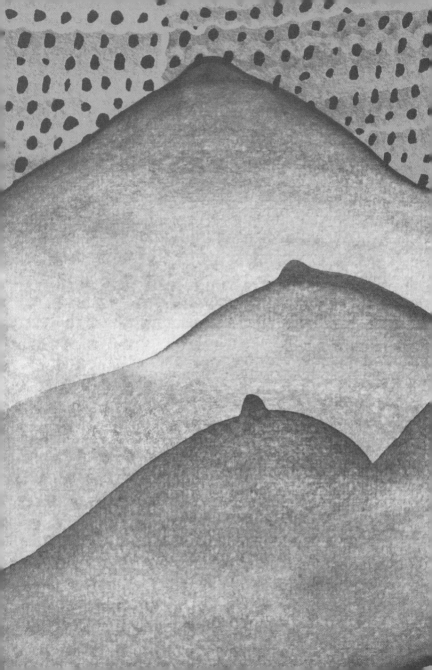

Part V. Pregnancy Health
Baby (on the) brain

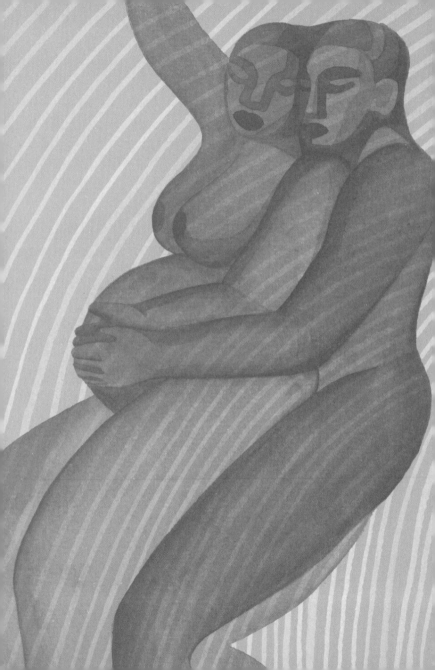

57. Make no assumptions about your fertility.

58. Use an app to track your cycles.

59. It may take you a year to get pregnant.

60. If you're younger than 35 and you're not pregnant after 12 months of trying, get thee to a gyno.

61. If you're 35 or older, give it only 6 months of trying before seeking help.

62. There's nothing wrong with needing help to get pregnant.

63. There's no wrong or unnatural way to deliver a baby.

64. Miscarriage is incredibly common.

65. The postpartum period can be rough.

66. Your body will change after you have a baby.

67. Having a C-section won't save your vagina.

68. Even if you're not having that much sex, you still need birth control after you have a baby.

69. Sex after pregnancy may be different.

57 Make no assumptions about your fertility.

I've delivered babies to two 12-year-olds in my career. I've also delivered the baby of a 51-year-old. If you're old enough to have a period, you're old enough to get pregnant. And until you've had 12 months without periods, you aren't truly in menopause and can still conceive. Your ovaries don't care if you're still a kid or if you have kids in college.

> **It's natural to worry about your fertility, even if you have zero intentions of getting pregnant soon. Or ever.**

But even though it's possible to get pregnant during half of your life, don't assume you'll always be able to get pregnant when you want to. I wish I could tell you there's an easy way to reassure yourself that your pregnancy parts are functioning as they should be. But there's no easy test for fertility. I'd never tell *anyone* to get pregnant before they're ready to become a parent, but if having a baby is incredibly important to you, don't put it off forever. After 35, getting pregnant becomes significantly more difficult and a bit riskier. Talk with your doctor about how best to stay healthy so you'll be able to get pregnant when you're ready.

Use an app to track your cycles.

58

You can increase your chances of pregnancy if you focus on having sex on days you can conceive. Use an app to follow your cycles for a few months. You generally ovulate 14 days before your period starts, so you only know for sure when you ovulated *after* your period comes. For example, if your cycles are typically 29 days long, you'll probably ovulate on Day 15 (where Day 1 is the first day of your period).

Your "fertile window" lasts from five days before ovulation to the day after. This is because sperm can live up to five days, waiting patiently for the egg to arrive. Once an egg is released from the ovary (ovulation), it can live for 24 hours. Your most fertile days are the two to three days before and the day of ovulation. Have sex every day to every other day during this time.

> **There are only about six days a month when sex can lead to pregnancy.**

Ovulation predictor kits from the drugstore can help you time sex for when you get the most buck for your bang. But if your cycles are very irregular, see your gyno for testing and advice.

59 It may take you a year to get pregnant.

After years of using birth control and worrying about an unplanned pregnancy, you may be galled to realize that you can't get pregnant as soon as you want to. In fact, your chance of conceiving in any given cycle is only about 25% (even lower if you're over 30). There's nothing wrong with you if it doesn't happen right away.

You can boost your chances of conception by:
- Tracking your periods and timing sex
- Having sex every day or every other day when you're fertile
- Avoiding lubricants that have been linked to decreased sperm motility and survival, including K-Y Jelly, K-Y Touch, Astroglide, olive oil, and saliva
- Not eating seafood high in mercury
- Quitting tobacco smoking and non-prescription drugs, including marijuana
- Not having more than two alcoholic drinks per day
- Reducing your caffeine consumption to below 200 mg daily (that's about 2 cups of coffee or 4 cans of cola)

There is no evidence that sexual position, orgasm or rest after intercourse increases your chance of pregnancy.

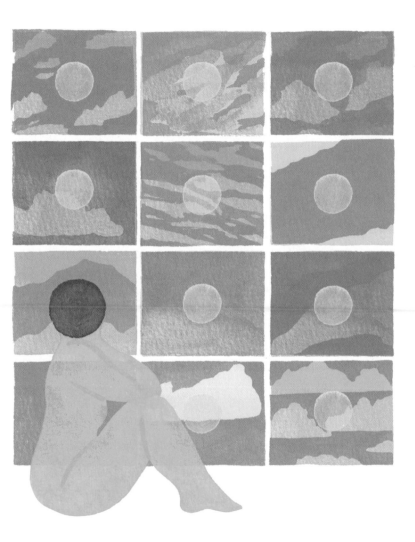

60 If you're younger than 35 and you're not pregnant after 12 months of trying, get thee to a gyno.

Most couples trying to get pregnant will succeed in the first six months. If you're hitting the 12-month mark and haven't gotten pregnant, that may be a sign that something is wrong. For example, you may have a blockage in your tubes or an ovulation problem, or your partner may have a low sperm count.

Some couples have a health history that puts them at increased risk of fertility challenges. Seek an evaluation from a gyno either before you try to get pregnant or after a few months of trying if any of the following apply to you or your partner:

- Irregular or no menstrual periods
- History of an STI or pelvic inflammatory disease (PID)
- Any surgery in your belly or pelvis
- Prior difficulty getting pregnant
- Known problems with testicles or genitals
- Hypospadias, where the opening of the urethra is not at the end of the penis
- Problems with ejaculation

If you're 35 or older, give it only 6 months of trying before seeking help. 61

No, 35 is not old — but it does make your eggs old. Egg quality and quantity decrease with age, and it becomes harder for everyone to conceive. If you're in your early 30s, you have about a 20% chance of conceiving each cycle. Your odds drop to about 5% each cycle by the time you reach 40. The sooner you reach out and get an evaluation by a gyno, the sooner you can get assistance to get pregnant. And even assistance has a lower success rate the older you get.

Your gyno may start your fertility evaluation or refer you to an infertility specialist, also known as a reproductive endocrinologist (REI). The first round of evaluation usually involves blood work to test your egg bank account (ovarian reserve) and ovulatory status, a special X-ray called a hystero-salpingogram (HSG) to check out your fallopian tubes and uterine cavity, and a semen analysis to look at your partner's sperm count and health.

Additional testing may include even more blood tests to screen for diseases, and genetic testing for you and your partner. It can be scary to undergo this much testing. But knowing what's going on with your body gives you either hope that you're healthy or a direction for treatment.

62 There's nothing wrong with needing help to get pregnant.

Some people feel like failures when they can't get pregnant on their own. Maybe they dreamed of noticing that their period was late, then taking a pregnancy test and being surprised and overjoyed at the results. The way your body works in union with your partner to start to grow a whole new human is a marvel.

It's no less marvelous when a little science and technology is needed. Assisted reproduction techniques include:

- Medications to increase your chance of ovulation
- Delivering sperm right into your uterus (often known as artificial insemination)
- In vitro fertilization (IVF)

These techniques have helped to form families that otherwise wouldn't have existed. They're especially crucial for couples who don't have all the necessary parts — sperm, eggs, and a uterus — to make a baby on their own.

Of course, there are other ways to build a family, including surrogacy and adoption. But many people dream of passing on their father's eyes or their mother's curly hair to a child of their own. If giving birth to a baby is your priority, it's OK to get help.

There's no wrong or unnatural way to deliver a baby.

63

Sure, pregnant people are often able to deliver a baby through the vagina, without medication. But deliveries don't always go as you've planned — just like you're not always able to get pregnant like you planned or avoid unexpected complications during the pregnancy. Despite birthing classes and breathing practice, you may be walloped by the pain of labor and decide to get an epidural after all. And if your labor isn't going well or the baby is refusing to come out or is in an awkward or backward (breech) position, a cesarean section may be the best thing to keep you both healthy.

There is no shame in getting through your delivery by any means necessary. Doctors define a successful delivery as one in which both the baby and parent get to leave the hospital alive and well. It is *not* a failure to need an epidural or a C-section during your delivery. They may not be part of the "natural" delivery you planned on, but you know what has historically been natural? Dying in childbirth, or the baby dying. I'm grateful that modern medicine has evolved to save more delivering persons and their babies than ever before.

64 Miscarriage is incredibly common.

Even in our share-everything, post-it-online culture, many people are not open about losing a pregnancy. But miscarriage happens to 1 out of every 3 or 4 pregnancies.

Most pregnancy losses, in the first trimester, happen due to an unpreventable and untreatable genetic problem with the pregnancy. Until recently, these miscarriages were virtually undetectable, noticed only as a late period. Because of cheap and super-accurate home pregnancy tests, more of these early miscarriages are being detected, leading to grief and worry about what having a miscarriage means.

Other kinds of losses are spoken about even less. The death of a baby in the third trimester is called a stillbirth, and doctors can't always tell why it happens. An ectopic pregnancy is life-threatening because it implants outside the uterus (in the fallopian tube, cervix, or C-section scar). Since an ectopic pregnancy can't be moved into the uterus, it must be removed from your body. And the strange-sounding molar pregnancy needs careful monitoring after removal because it could lead to cancer.

Any loss may be devastating—or a relief, if it was a pregnancy you weren't ready for. Either way, know that a loss doesn't affect your ability to have a healthy baby someday, if you want one.

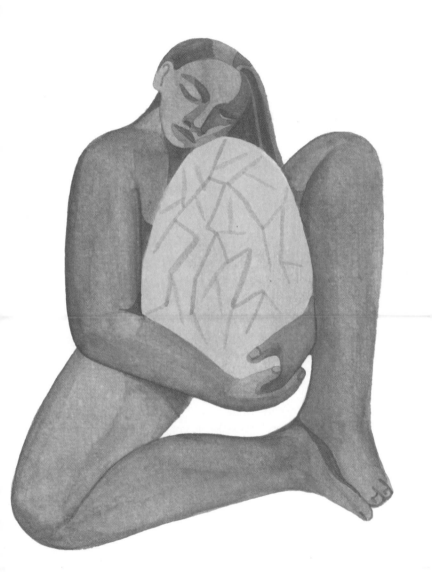

65 The postpartum period can be rough.

Going through childbirth is an awesome experience that's as life-changing as everyone says it is. But it's also a trial by fire that can leave you feeling battered. You may be unprepared for the afterbirth pains and burning while you pee for the first few days after the baby is born. It's common to feel exhausted and winded for days, if not weeks. You may have sweating that soaks your clothes, especially at night. Even I was caught off-guard by how heavy the first post-baby period is (a nurse had to point out that I had bled through my scrubs). And sadly, it's natural for the extra lush hair on your head that you grew in pregnancy to fall out in the months following childbirth.

Your body is amazing in how it heals. Your puffy face and legs will return to their pre-pregnancy size. If you delivered through the vagina, cuts or tears will heal, most often without scarring. If you've had a C-section, the scar will fade with time. And the baby blues — mood swings, anxiety, or irritability — that up to 70% of people experience should fade away by the time your baby is 2 weeks old. You've got this.

Your body will change after you have a baby.

66

When you've just grown and birthed a whole human, there's no other way around it — that's going to lead to some changes.

While there's a lot of information about what to expect with pregnancy and childbirth, you may be less prepared for the other changes that might happen. You'll get stretch marks over your breasts, belly, hips and thighs. Your belly may have a gap between your abs (diastasis recti), and a lower belly pooch. A weakening of your pelvic floor muscles may mean you'll leak urine when you laugh or cough. Vaginal dryness is common, due to a drop in hormone levels. And hemorrhoids (swollen veins in and around the anus) may make anal sex painful. Even your feet may change, becoming larger, and your mood may be all over the place for a few months.

> **You can't avoid post-pregnancy changes in your breasts by not breastfeeding. It's the change in the weight of your breasts that makes them saggy.**

Try to see these changes in a positive way: They're marks on a body that did an *amazing* thing, a body that continues to protect and care for the baby you had. These changes are a sign of strength, and you should be proud of what your body accomplished.

67 Having a C-section won't save your vagina.

Many pregnant people dread the thought of what giving birth will do to their vagina. They've heard horror stories about leaking urine (incontinence) and worse, the bulging of the walls of the vagina out the opening (prolapse). Some people worry so much about delivery that they request a cesarean section, thinking that it will protect their vagina from harm.

Sadly, there's no getting around the fact that pregnancy can do a number on your body. When it comes to your post-delivery vaginal health, it's not just the delivery that influences how quickly your body heals. Carrying the weight of the baby in your body for nine months, with the baby's head bearing down, creates the risk of loosening of your pelvic floor muscles, no matter how the baby is born. Certainly, a C-section avoids additional trauma to your vagina, but it too has consequences. A post-C-section scarred uterus is never as strong as one without a scar, and you'll have risks of placenta problems in future pregnancies, along with scar tissue formation in your pelvis outside the uterus. If your labor lets you deliver vaginally, it truly is the safest way to go for your body.

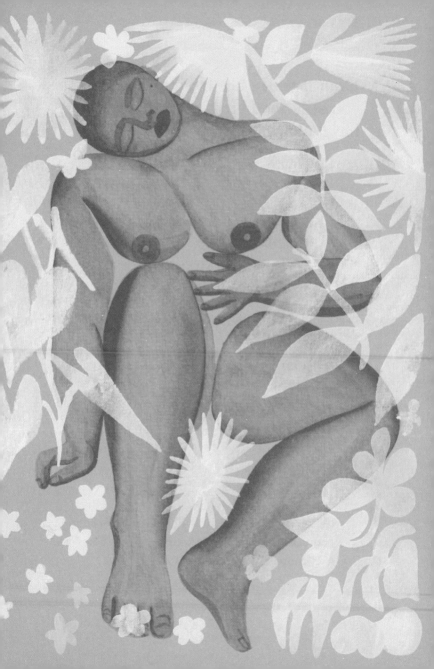

68 Even if you're not having that much sex, you still need birth control after you have a baby.

It's understandable if you think you can't get pregnant again shortly after you give birth to a baby. You might think that growing an entire human being would earn you some relief from worrying about an unwanted pregnancy. But the surprising truth is that you can ovulate as soon as *25 days* after you deliver. That means you can get pregnant with a 1-month-old infant in the cradle. Breastfeeding only works as birth control if you're solely nursing (not pumping) and even then, only for six months, and only if your periods haven't returned.

Since there's no justice in the universe around pregnancy, even one night of sex when the baby is still new can result in the conception of Junior's sibling. All it takes is sex once at the right (or wrong) time to get pregnant. So, if you're not interested in having your pregnancies thiiiiis close together, make sure your gyno has set you up with postpartum contraception. This way, when the mood strikes and the baby's sleeping, you'll be prepared.

It's healthiest to wait 18 months before becoming pregnant again, to allow your body to recover and heal from the first pregnancy.

Sex after pregnancy may be different. 69

Your body and mood may feel different after you have a baby. Your pelvic floor muscles may be stretched, bruised or torn. Your falling estrogen levels may lead to less vaginal elasticity and lubrication. Sex may be uncomfortable or even painful at first. And when you're exhausted from caring for a newborn, your libido may not be what it used to be pre-baby.

Waiting for penetrative sex until four to six weeks after giving birth, no matter how you delivered the baby, allows your body to heal (though orgasms are just fine). Give yourself time to get your sexual self back. If you're not able to get in the mood for sex weeks or months after delivery and this distresses you, be alert for signs of postpartum depression.

If you have a partner, you can keep up your intimacy by spending time together without the baby, even if it's just for a few minutes at the start and the end of the day. Consider scheduling sexy time, working around the baby's sleep schedule or when you can get a sitter. If you haven't used lubricant before, now is an excellent time to try one. After a while, sex may be even better than it was before.

Conception Checkup

When you're ready to try to get pregnant:

- ☐ Start taking prenatal vitamins, which can be over the counter or prescription.
- ☐ Time sex to your "fertile window" each month.
- ☐ Use lubricants that don't affect sperm, including Pre-Seed, ConceivEase, canola oil and mineral oil.
- ☐ Avoid seafood high in mercury, including king mackerel (kingfish), marlin, northern pike, orange roughy, shark, swordfish, tilefish, and ahi and bigeye tuna.
- ☐ Toss the tobacco products, and avoid all non-prescription drugs including marijuana.
- ☐ Don't have more than two alcoholic drinks per day.
- ☐ Cut back on your caffeine intake, sticking to less than 200 mg a day, or fewer than 2 cups of coffee or 4 cans of cola a day.
- ☐ Let your doctors know you're trying to get pregnant so they can review your health history and medications to make sure you're set to conceive.

Ask Your Doctor...

I encourage you to ask your doctor any of these questions:

- ☐ My periods are irregular. Can you help me figure out my fertile window?
- ☐ Does pregnancy pose any risk for me, based on my medical history?
- ☐ I haven't gotten pregnant after 6 to 12 months of trying. What can I do?
- ☐ Can you recommend a urologist for my partner to see for evaluation?
- ☐ Do you or your partners offer fertility treatments?
- ☐ Can we do testing to figure out why I had a miscarriage?
- ☐ What kind of birth control can I use after the baby is born?
- ☐ Can you show me how to do a Kegel exercise?

Afterword

Now that you've reached the end of this book, what happens next is in your hands. How do you feel about your body? About your sexual health? About the steps you want to take — or *don't* want to take? With whom — and how — you want to share your body? What glimmers of insight from this book will you carry with you?

At a minimum, I hope you understand your body even just a little better than you did. That you have a better sense of what your body's telling you — and how to know when *not* to worry about what you feel or see. I also hope you feel more able and encouraged to make the choices that are right for you — and confident to ask for help when you need it. Your health care team is there for you, ready to help you do what feels best for your health and well-being.

But maybe most important, I hope that you can see your body in a way that leads to acceptance, and even peace. Your parts are part of you, not strangers or, even worse, your enemies. You only get one body, and it's your partner for life. Now that you know more, try to see yourself in a stronger, positive light — and cherish your body for the gift that it is.

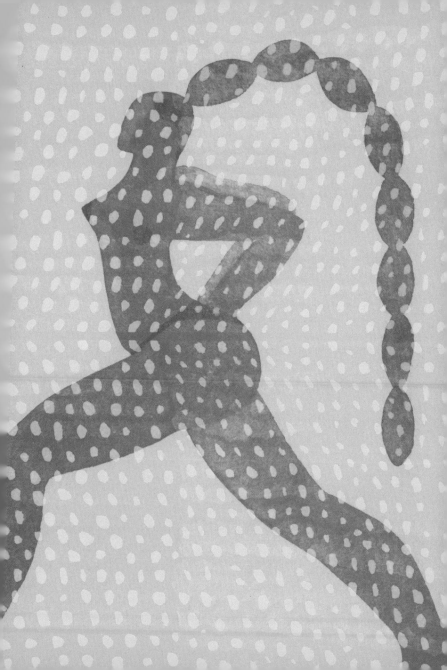

The author wishes to thank the team at Mayo Clinic Press (in particular Stephanie K. Vaughan), her family for their encouragement (especially her husband, Chad White), her early readers for their input, and her patients for their trust.

MAYO CLINIC PRESS
200 First St. SW
Rochester, MN 55905

http://mcpress.MayoClinic.org

The information in this book is true and complete to the best of our knowledge. This book is intended as an informative guide for those wishing to learn more about health issues. It is not intended to replace, countermand or conflict with advice given to you by your own physician. The ultimate decision concerning your care should be made between you and your doctor. Information in this book is offered with no guarantees.

The author and publisher disclaim all liability in connection with the use of this publication. The views expressed are the author's personal views, and do not necessarily reflect the policy or position of Mayo Clinic.

To stay informed about Mayo Clinic Press, please subscribe to our free e-newsletter at http://mcpress.MayoClinic.org or follow us on social media.

For bulk sales to employers, member groups and health-related companies, contact Mayo Clinic at SpecialSalesMayoBooks@mayo.edu.

Proceeds from the sale of every book benefit important medical education and research at Mayo Clinic.

Managing editor: Stephanie K. Vaughan
Production design: North Market Street Graphics
Illustrations: Monica Ramos

ISBN 978-1-893005-85-3
Library of Congress Control Number: 2021949472

Printed in China